GUT BACTERIA ROLES IN DEPRESSION

The factors, effects, and therapy of gut bacteria.

By

Dr. DOUGLAS JASON

GUT BACTERIA ROLES IN DEPRESSION

Copyright © (DR DOUGLAS JASON) 2022. All rights reserved

Before this document is duplicated or reproduced in any manner, the publisher's consent must be gained.

Therefore, the contents within can neither be stored electronically, transferred, nor kept in a database. Neither in part nor in full can the document be copied, scanned, faxed, or retained without approval from the publisher or creator.

GUT BACTERIA ROLES IN DEPRESSION

GUT BACTERIA ROLES IN DEPRESSION

TABLE OF CONTENT

ABOUT THE AUTHOR

INTRODUCTION

GUT BACTERIA ROLES IN DEPRESSION

TABLE OF CONTENT

GUT BACTERIA ROLES IN DEPRESSION

The factors, effects, and therapy of gut bacteria.

INTRODUCTION

CHAPTER 1
GENETIC FACTOR.

CHAPTER 2

GUT BACTERIA ROLES IN DEPRESSION

THE PART OF BACTERIA.

CHAPTER 3
WHAT ARE THE CLINICAL IMPLICATIONS?

CHAPTER 4
discusses the brain's glutamate transmission.

CHAPTER 5
Therapies for depression of the gut-brain.

GUT BACTERIA ROLES IN DEPRESSION

CHAPTER 6
How can someone tell whether they need therapy?

GUT BACTERIA ROLES IN DEPRESSION

ABOUT THE AUTHOR

Dr. Douglas Jason is a certified dietician who has a strong passion for wellness and a big eagerness to help people all over the world. He uses healthy food, herbs, spices, and other useful tools to help mankind realize its overall goal of optimum health.

GUT BACTERIA ROLES IN DEPRESSION

INTRODUCTION

cause of disability in the world (WHO).
According to research, ethnic differences in depression symptom severity and the gut microbiota's potential role in depressive disorders are both present.
13 various species of gut bacteria have now been linked to the symptoms of depression, according to studies from the UK and the Netherlands.
A recent study, appearing in Nature Communications, demonstrates how gut bacteria may contribute to

GUT BACTERIA ROLES IN DEPRESSION

sadness by producing neurotransmitters like glutamate and serotonin.

Chronic sadness, emptiness, or the inability to experience pleasure are all symptoms of depression. Although the causes of depression are not fully understood, it is likely that several elements, which we will discuss in this book, are involved:

GUT BACTERIA ROLES IN DEPRESSION

CHAPTER 1

GENETIC FACTOR.

changes in the brain's neurotransmitter levels, environmental influences such as trauma exposure, psychological factors, and social factors

What did the research reveal? Investigators from Oxford Population Health and colleagues from the Netherlands examined the association between the variety and

GUT BACTERIA ROLES IN DEPRESSION

makeup of the gut microbiota and depressive symptoms in this study.

They looked at data from the Rotterdam Study's 1,133 participants. They made certain to account for medication use and lifestyle factors in their analysis. For example, they only took into account people who weren't using antidepressants.

To estimate changes in the gut microbiota that are a result of the depression or the medicine rather

GUT BACTERIA ROLES IN DEPRESSION

than a cause, this precaution was taken.

Numerous bacteria were found to possibly play a role in how people generate neurotransmitters, notably those like glutamate that has been related to depression.

Using information from the HELIUS trial, an additional observational study, the researchers subsequently repeated and validated these findings.

GUT BACTERIA ROLES IN DEPRESSION

One day, new medicines for ailments like depression could be created thanks to the findings of this study.

GUT BACTERIA ROLES IN DEPRESSION

CHAPTER 2

THE PART OF BACTERIA.

The study's senior research associate and author, Dr. Najaf Amin, emphasized the important findings by stating that the team had "discovered 13 species of bacteria [12 genera and one family] related with depression."

While Coprococcus, Lachnospiraceae UCG001, Ruminococcusgauvreauii group,

GUT BACTERIA ROLES IN DEPRESSION

Eubacterium ventricose, Subdoligranulum, Ruminococcaceae (UCG002, UCG003, UCG005), and [the] family Ruminococcaceae were slighter abundant in individuals with higher symptoms of depression, she explained, "Eggerthella, Hungatella, Sellimonas, and Lachnoclos

These bacteria are known to affect depression by participating in the metabolism of some important chemicals, such as glutamate and butyrate.

GUT BACTERIA ROLES IN DEPRESSION

CHAPTER 3

WHAT ARE THE CLINICAL IMPLICATIONS?

According to Dr. Amin, "big and meticulous research on the relationship between the gut microbiome and depression was lacking." Such investigations, in her words, "provide biomarkers and therapeutic targets for the disease,

GUT BACTERIA ROLES IN DEPRESSION

and are the first step towards understanding the pathophysiology."

"Since nutrition, in particular, is largely responsible for determining gut microbiome, once causality is proved, the therapy would be as straightforward as modifying diet or taking probiotics," she pointed out.

"Additionally, depression is a condition that is both underdiagnosed and overdiagnosed. A biomarker will make it possible to assess depression objectively, which is

GUT BACTERIA ROLES IN DEPRESSION

currently impossible, enhancing diagnosis, according to Dr. Amin.

We know that the microbiome influences our mood, according to Dr. Neil Paulvin, a New York-based expert in anti-aging and regenerative medicine who was not involved in the study.

"Neurotransmitters including nana, serotonin, and norepinephrine are produced by the microbiota. The future of mental health includes this, he continued.

GUT BACTERIA ROLES IN DEPRESSION

"We need to identify the precise mix of gut bacteria that is beneficial and detrimental for anxiety. For instance, which bacteria can alter serotonin to aid with depression, which bacteria can activate GABA [gamma-aminobutyric acid, a neurotransmitter] to help with anxiety, and whether fecal microbiota transplant will be a solution for depression and anxiety.

Dr. Paulvin emphasized that there are now being developed tablet

GUT BACTERIA ROLES IN DEPRESSION

psychobiotics (probiotics that alter mood).

Dr. Paulvin stated, "We are currently cultivating the knowledge to construct programs in the future."

GUT BACTERIA ROLES IN DEPRESSION

CHAPTER 4

discusses the brain's glutamate transmission.

This is a very well-done study that controlled for several potentially interfering variables, and in doing so, demonstrated the role of certain gut microbiome species in providing chemical modulators that are known to have both direct and indirect effects on brain chemistry involved

GUT BACTERIA ROLES IN DEPRESSION

in cognitive and emotional function, according to Dr. James Giordano, Pellegrino lecturer of Neurology and Biochemistry at Georgetown University Medical Center, who was also not involved in this research.

In particular, he said, "it has been demonstrated that the gut species Eggerthella and Eubacterium ventriosum create butyrate, a key precursor molecule to GABA, a brain neurotransmitter that serves in the regulatory regulation of glutamate.

GUT BACTERIA ROLES IN DEPRESSION

Additionally, it was discovered that these species produce serotonin, which affects the gut-brain axis and enteric nervous system directly. Serotonin levels and activity in the brain are therefore crucial for aspects of cognitive, emotional, and behavioral function.

The gut microbiome's contribution to GABA- and serotonin-mediated control of brain glutamate activity (primarily via modulation of the

GUT BACTERIA ROLES IN DEPRESSION

vagus nerve) may be a key mechanism for preserving mental health. Overactive glutamate transmission in the brain has been shown to contribute to several symptoms of depressive and anxiety disorders.

The study also showed that specific other species of the gut [bacteria] can have negative impacts on the enteric nervous system, gut-brain axis, brain chemistry, and the expression of depression and

GUT BACTERIA ROLES IN DEPRESSION

anxiety disorders' signs and symptoms.

As a result, Dr. Giordano said, "overgrowth of these species, as well as undergrowth or under activity of beneficial species, can produce local and systemic inflammatory states, which can disrupt the biochemical and physiological stability of the brain, and contribute to the development and exacerbation of neuro-psychiatric conditions."

GUT BACTERIA ROLES IN DEPRESSION

It is feasible to change the makeup of these bacterial populations, according to Dr. Amin. Utilizing prebiotics and probiotics makes this possible. For instance, consuming high-fiber foods like fresh fruits, whole grains, and vegetables can change the bacterium that produces butyrate.

The findings of this study, in Dr. Giordano's words, "provide a crucial takeaway message that gut health via [the] stability of the gut

GUT BACTERIA ROLES IN DEPRESSION

microbiota is important to maintaining brain functions that are engaged in thought, emotion, and behavior."

According to him, "the gut-brain axis and the growing understanding of the gut microbiota strengthen that the cautious use of pre-and probiotics can be of help in supporting both gut and brain health."

GUT BACTERIA ROLES IN DEPRESSION

GUT BACTERIA ROLES IN DEPRESSION

CHAPTER 5

Therapies for depression of the gut-brain.

A person may participate in a variety of therapies, such as:

Cognitive-behavioral therapy (CBT): According to the American Psychological Association (APA), CBT is successful in treating a variety of problems, including eating disorders, anxiety, and depression.

Talking or interpersonal therapy: According to the National Health Service (NHS) of the United Kingdom, interpersonal therapy aids depressed individuals in recognizing and resolving relationship issues.

Emotion-focused therapy: According to a current 2018 study, this kind of therapy may be able to help those who are suffering from disorders like depression, trauma, and social anxiety.

Group therapy: A person participates in a session with others

GUT BACTERIA ROLES IN DEPRESSION

who have gone through similar things to express feelings and provide support to one another. A trained mental health care provider usually conducts sessions.

In therapy sessions, therapists employ a variety of strategies to assist their patients, including talking treatments, aid in managing negative thoughts, social interaction, and mindfulness exercises.

GUT BACTERIA ROLES IN DEPRESSION

CHAPTER 6

How can someone tell whether they need therapy?

According to the National Institute of Mental Health, self-care activities can help those who are depressed or having trouble falling asleep. These consist of:

Exercise chatting with a friend eating healthfully meditating

GUT BACTERIA ROLES IN DEPRESSION

However, if a person's symptoms don't go away or last for more than two weeks, or if they encounter any of the following, they might think about speaking with a therapist:

inability to focus, lack of motivation, and thoughts of harming oneself or others
diminished appetite
feeling depressed or blue, frustrated, or anxious

How to locate a cheap therapist

GUT BACTERIA ROLES IN DEPRESSION

When seeking out reasonably priced therapy, there are several factors to take into account:

Cost and insurance: Some businesses use subscription-based services, allowing customers to cancel at any time. Although some mental health therapies are not covered by some insurance plans, health insurance could help to lower overall costs. Therefore, it is best to check with an insurer or employer to determine if they are covered before going to therapy.

GUT BACTERIA ROLES IN DEPRESSION

Reviews: One can examine a company's reviews and reputation using unbiased services like the Better Business Bureau (BBB) or Trustpilot.

Credentials: Some counseling services let clients view the credentials, expertise, and specializations of their therapists. This might make it possible to calculate costs.

Usefulness: A lot of therapists provide online sessions via video, phone, or instant message chats, which people may find to be more economical.

GUT BACTERIA ROLES IN DEPRESSION

Some of the top low-cost solutions for internet therapy
Here are a few businesses that provide internet counseling sessions at reasonable prices.

Please be aware that the book's author has not used any of these goods. The knowledge offered is entirely based on research.

Prices and reviews were accurate when this book was published.

GUT BACTERIA ROLES IN DEPRESSION

BetterHelp
Individual, couple, and teen counseling sessions are available from BetterHelp. For the platform to match a user with a therapist, a questionnaire must be filled out by the user.

A person can communicate with a therapist over the phone, via video chat, or via instant messaging.

Additionally, BetterHelp provides:

GUT BACTERIA ROLES IN DEPRESSION

group sessions with flexible scheduling and digital worksheets to aid in the therapeutic process
The platform collaborates with certified counselors, clinical social workers, marital and family therapists, and psychologists.

The cost of counseling ranges from $60 to $90 per week, and clients have the option of leaving at any moment. BetterHelp services are

GUT BACTERIA ROLES IN DEPRESSION

not often covered by health insurance programs, though.

BetterHelp has a BBB grade of A and an overall rating of 4.1 out of 5. Reviews claim that sessions are very convenient and that therapists are sympathetic and helpful.

The therapists at Amwell Amwell offer therapy for a range of mental health issues, including:

GUT BACTERIA ROLES IN DEPRESSION

sleeplessness panic attacks
relationship problems
grieving, social anxiety
A client can select a therapist who holds a Master's or Ph.D. in their specialty. Prices typically range from $109 to 129, and they depend on the qualifications and experience of the therapist.

Additionally, the business employs doctors and psychiatrists who may write prescriptions and oversee urgent care.

GUT BACTERIA ROLES IN DEPRESSION

Amwell works with numerous insurers, so a person should check their coverage by contacting their insurer or employer.

Amwell receives 3.1 out of 5 stars from Trustpilot users who also note that the cost can be greater than in-person appointments and that not all medications are prescribed by the doctors there. However, some said that they swiftly obtained a diagnosis and treatment plan.

GUT BACTERIA ROLES IN DEPRESSION

ReGain

The ReGain platform connects users with qualified mental healthcare professionals to provide treatment sessions for both individuals and couples.

Couples counseling requires that both participants be in the same place; ReGain does not currently provide live three-way sessions.

GUT BACTERIA ROLES IN DEPRESSION

All written material is saved in the company's chat room once users log in for future reference, but only the counselor and one or more partners have access.

ReGain has a subscription-based pricing structure, with weekly sessions ranging from $60 to $90. Private medical insurers are not now a part of the company's business.

On Trustpilot, the business has received a rating of 1.8 stars out of

GUT BACTERIA ROLES IN DEPRESSION

5, with fewer positive remarks referencing paying a month in advance and that the service was unable to schedule an appointment with a counselor. There were no favorable reviews available at the time this article was published.

Medical on Demand
A platform with a focus on physical and mental health issues is called Doctor on Demand.

GUT BACTERIA ROLES IN DEPRESSION

It provides treatment sessions with qualified licensed mental health professionals who can assist people with stress, trauma, anxiety, and depression. A psychiatrist who offers treatment sessions and, if required, prescribes restricted drugs can also be consulted. People might need to make an in-person appointment with their doctor if they need a prescription for a controlled substance, such as an anxiety medication.

GUT BACTERIA ROLES IN DEPRESSION

Prices for Doctor on Demand vary from $130 to $300 depending on the length of the appointment or the type of therapist.

During the registration process, one can determine if telehealth consultations with Doctors on Demand are covered by their insurer.

GUT BACTERIA ROLES IN DEPRESSION

www.ingramcontent.com/pod-product-compliance
Lightning Source LLC
Chambersburg PA
CBHW050316220526
45465CB00005B/2019